How

Live Green

Guide to Getting Started With Green Living so You Can Protect Your Health, Your Home and the Environment While Also Saving Money

By Jeremy Nash

© **Copyright 2021 - All rights reserved.**

The content contained within this book may not be reproduced, duplicated or transmitted without direct written permission from the author or the publisher.

Under no circumstances will any blame or legal responsibility be held against the publisher or author for any damages, reparation, or monetary loss due to the information contained within this book. Either directly or indirectly.

Legal Notice:

This book is copyright protected. This book is only for personal use. You cannot amend, distribute, sell, use, quote or paraphrase any part, or the content within this book, without the consent of the author or publisher.

Disclaimer Notice:

Please note the information contained within this document is for educational and entertainment purposes only. All effort has been executed to present accurate, up to date and reliable, complete information. No warranties of any kind are declared or implied. Readers acknowledge that the author is not engaging in the rendering of legal, financial, medical or professional advice. The content within this book has been derived from various sources. Please consult a licensed professional before attempting any techniques outlined in this book.

By reading this document, the reader agrees that under no

circumstances is the author responsible for any losses, direct or indirect, which are incurred as a result of the use of information contained within this document, including, but not limited to, —errors, omissions, or inaccuracies.

Contents

Chapter 1: What Is Green Living 1
   The Importance of Living Green 2
Chapter 2: Recycling 6
   Precycling 7
   Paper 10
   Cardboard Boxes 10
   Glass 12
   Metal Cans 14
   Plastic 15
Chapter 3: Water 18
Chapter 4: Your House 20
   The Kitchen Space 22
      Utilize a Good Detergent 23
      Utilize Green Cleansing Products 24
      Aerate Your Faucets 27
      Reusable Containers 28
      Water Heating Units 28
      Ditch the Styrofoam 29
   The Restroom 30
      Showers 31
      Toilets 32
   The Bedroom 34
      Pillowcases and Sheets 34
      Comforters 34

Pillows 35

Curtains and Drapes 35

Chapter 5: Eating Green and Healthy 36

Chapter 6: Clothes 39

Purchasing Green Clothes 39

Looking After Green Clothes 40

Chapter 7: Transport 42

Maintaining the Tires 44

Transportation Alternatives 45

Conclusion 47

Thank you for buying this book and I hope that you will find it useful. If you will want to share your thoughts on this book, you can do so by leaving a review on the Amazon page, it helps me out a lot.

Chapter 1: What Is Green Living

Just what is green living? Actually, it boils down to one basic idea: the earth's resources have to be renewed at the identical rate that we're utilizing them. That indicates taking care of the environment by taking actions to save it.

If you begin taking a look at all the various types of resources we have - wildlife, fossil fuels, oceans, forests, and air - you may see that all of it is connected. Due to the fact that holds true, what we utilize today affects what we will have accessible for usage down the road.

Green living has to do with altering choices, choices which will definitely make our world and us better off. We have a window of possibility that we may utilize to begin recovery and restoring and fixing our environment, from rivers and oceans to meadows and rain forests.

The Importance of Living Green

Edgar Mitchell, an Apollo 14 astronaut, said that in the 20th century, we advanced with the power of technology and science into a non-sustainable civilization - our most instant risk is what we are doing to ourselves due to our lack of knowledge and unwillingness as people and countries to face the ecological issues. To challenge the excesses of our civilization, of contamination and nonrenewable resources, dangers of trash accumulating and our oceans being contaminated. The huge issue has to do with our patterns of consumption; more is better and cash is the only genuine worth that may make you pleased. We need to alter our thinking patterns and our ways if we are to make it through.

it took mother earth 100 million years to develop the energy that we, as a world, utilize today in one year? I'm certain that you do understand that cancer, asthma, and lots of other illnesses are more common today than ever in history.

Lots of professionals link the boost in illnesses to the modifications in our environment.

Fortunately, we do have time to start to alter our environment. Every one of us has to be responsible for our decisions. Every one of us chooses things daily that may have an effect on the whole world. Much of these options we take for granted, like driving to work rather than taking public transportation, or purchasing packaged food rather than natural or fresh. Choices such as this might appear small, however, they are anything but, specifically when multiplied by the billions of individuals.

Green living can assist the world, and it can likewise assist you in lots of other manners:

- Sparing cash - We are used to consuming a lot more than we require. If we consume what we, in fact, require, whether it's water or electrical power or clothing or some other product, we are going to spare cash. Specific instance? For each 1 ° central heating is cranked up, the costs grow by

8%. Here's another: Placing a water filled bottle within the toilet tank reduces water usage per flush by 33%.

- Community assistance - In case we support the shops in our community which promote green living, we assist those organizations to remain profitable, we act in socially and ecologically accountable manner, and we send out a message to less savvy businesses that they have to do things differently.

- Health benefits - If we live green via walking or biking more frequently rather than driving and through more greener options with the food we consume, it is going to enhance our health in every manner.

Many individuals do not understand how to start living green, however, it isn't tough whatsoever. It's actually a matter of making different decisions about how you do things daily. By the end of this guide, you are going to have all the details you require to start with green living in each aspect of your life.

Chapter 2: Recycling

Individuals are typically acquainted with the word recycling. If you can't repurpose or recycle things, recycling is the next choice. Recycling includes gathering things that are no longer helpful in their existing shape and processing them, their parts, or a few of their parts into basic materials from which brand-new products are created.

Have you ever questioned simply how reliable recycling is? Here's a figure: recycling aluminum, steel, lead, copper, plastics, and paper may spare between 60% and 90% of the energy it requires to make brand-new items from these things. Recycling not just decreases garbage that goes to incinerators and landfills, however, it likewise decreases the quantity of greenhouse gases launched into the atmosphere. EPA data for 2005 states that recycling stopped the release of 79 million tons of carbon into the air. That is approximately as much as it is generated every year by 40 million automobiles.

You may see that recycling is far more desirable than merely tossing a thing in the garbage. Cities and states are ending up being greener constantly and making it simpler for everybody to recycle.

Precycling

While we have actually all become aware of recycling, you might not recognize the word "precycling." This principle was introduced in 1989 in Berkeley, California, where the city started an initiative to motivate customers to purchase food packaged in recyclable or eco-friendly materials. To put it simply, we recycle things after we have actually purchased and utilized them, however, we precycle while we're shopping.

This might be the simplest means to live green. If we make the right purchasing decisions, we may stop undesirable things from entering into our system.

- Every American utilizes around 200 pounds of plastic annually. About 65 pounds of that is disposed of as quickly as the bundle is opened.

- 30% of all plastics are utilized for product wrapping, and Americans squander 3 million plastic bottles each hour.

- Wrapping waste represents one-third of all trash in the landfills in America.

- Roughly 5 million tons (the majority of all plastics we get rid of annually) are wrapping.

We may minimize these numbers quickly. Here are several things you may do, beginning today, to reduce wrapping waste with precycling:

- Purchase in cardboard containers.

- Purchase cereal in boxes crafted from recycled cardboard. Those boxes are grey on the within.

- Purchase wholesale - it's less expensive and utilizes very little packaging.

- We frequently have an option of purchasing drinks in aluminum or glass containers instead of plastic. Pick aluminum or glass due to the fact that it's simple to recycle. The identical concept applies to purchasing dressings, sauces, spreads, baby food, and other products.

- When you have an option, stay clear of purchasing products in plastic containers.

Here's an incredible fact to remember: if 10% of Americans bought items with less plastic wrapping simply 10% of the time, we might get rid of 144 million pounds of plastic and lower commercial contamination.

See, that isn't so difficult. In the remainder of this guide, we are going to have a look at other simple and crucial methods to start with green living.

Paper

Technology might be resolving this issue for us on a big level given that increasingly more individuals are utilizing smartphones and computers to get their news. In case you still get newspapers, do not toss them out with the trash any longer. Take them to your recycling center. Pile them up till you have a big stack, and turn it into a practice to do so.

Americans utilize 50 million tons of paper every year, and that implies we chop down more than 850 million trees. If we create brand-new paper from recycled paper, it would utilize 40% less energy than creating paper from trees. The associated air contamination is decreased by 90%.

Cardboard Boxes

Cardboard boxes, specifically corrugated ones, could be cheaply recycled. You may recycle them into more cardboard, paper towels, toilet paper, manufactured wood, furniture, feline litter, pressboard, and other things.

Repurposing and Reusing:

- Reuse paper that's just been utilized on one side. You may do this by using paper from your printer, utilizing the other side for outlines. You can utilize it for a variety of things, such as notes, grocery lists, and so on.

- Utilize gift bags and wrapping paper once again – be cautious how you store it, and wrapping paper could be used again fairly often. In case you can't utilize all of it, you may be able to chop off the unusable part and utilize the remainder. Cut down all welcoming cards to create gift tags.

- Liners - utilize old magazines and newspapers to line drawers, boxes and kitty litter trays.

Another method to take a look at sparing paper is not to utilize it whatsoever. We can use cloth objects instead of paper objects in a number of methods. For example, attempt utilizing fabric shopping bags for your groceries. They're recyclable, and they keep lots of paper and plastic out of landfills annually. How about the paper towels which the majority of us utilize generously? Utilize cloth towels for kitchen area clean-ups, and you get to keep that additional paper out of the landfills and spare yourself some cash too.

Glass

Annually we get rid of 30 billion glass containers and bottles. Most glass is constructed from 3 standard parts: white sand, lime, and soda. These products are warmed to around 2500 ° F. Then the mix is cooled to 1800 ° F. The procedure requires 7600 BTUs of energy to generate a single glass piece.

These shocking stats may amaze you:

- All glass containers and bottles could be recycled.

- Glass created from recycled glass rather than basic material decreases associated air contamination by 20% and water contamination by half.

- It may take 3000 years for a glass container to disintegrate.

However, you'll enjoy the fact that all the glass you give for recycling really is recycled. This suggests consuming less natural resources. It likewise suggests much less waste - every ton of glass created makes 390 pounds of waste.

Lots of communities nowadays provide recycling bins to the houses. In case this does not apply to your community, you may quickly recycle glass by having a box for it in a practical location such as on your back porch or in your kitchen area. It's simple to do and a simple practice to start. Do not forget that you may find brand-new methods to utilize old glass.

Metal Cans

Aluminum is the most plentiful metal in the world. Hard to believe that it wasn't found up until the 1820s. The aluminum drink can initially appeared in 1963, and today it's the single biggest usage of aluminum. A lot of beverage and food cans created from steel or aluminum are recyclable. You may recycle utilized aluminum foil as well.

An aluminum can that you toss out today might be discovered by your forefathers as much as 500 years from today. The energy conserved from one recycled aluminum can might run a TV for 3 hours. Creating aluminum from recycled aluminum utilizes 90% less energy as opposed to creating aluminum from the ground up.

You may earn money from recycling aluminum cans and other aluminum items. Can recycle devices are going to pay you a set quantity for every single pound of the cans you turn in. Recycle centers may pay you even nicer rates.

Plastic

Many plastics are recyclable, however, this is a little difficult due to the fact that there are 7 various plastic kinds. Every plastic product is coded with a triangle stamp with the number between 1 and 7 within it. The code normally shows up on the plastic item bottom. Plastics with the numbers 1 or 2 are most quickly recyclable.

Code 1 This is polyethylene terephthalate. It is utilized to create juice, soda, and toiletry bottles. It may be developed into carpets and shirt components.

Code 2 High-density polyethylene. It is utilized to create detergent bottles, milk containers, and bleach bottles. It may be developed into detergent bottles, fencing and binders.

Code 3 This is polyvinyl chloride. It is utilized to create mineral water and shampoo bottles, house piping and siding. It may be developed into brand-new home piping, siding, and other property components.

Code 4 This is low-density polyethylene. It is utilized to create trash, grocery, and bread bags. It could be developed into brand-new bags.

Code 5 This is polypropylene. It is utilized to create dairy and margarine tubs. It could be developed into milk crates and vehicle parts.

Code 6 This is polystyrene. It is utilized to create coffee cups, meal trays, and wrapping. It could be developed into CD trays and DVD cases.

Code 7 This consists of other plastics. They are utilized for ketchup bottles, and so on, and they could be developed into picnic and park benches.

Contact your regional provider regarding which plastics they accept for recycling. Purchase the items with those numbers if feasible. Likewise, attempt to decrease the plastic that you purchase and use plastic again if you can.

Chapter 3: Water

70% of the earth's surface consists of water. That seems like a lot, however, our supply of water is being threatened by reckless utilization and contamination. United Nation's stats state that the global absence of fresh water and appropriate sanitation is wiping out 5 million individuals a year.

Even with global warming and the emerging melting Polar ice caps, the majority of that water enters into the salted sea. We discard big quantities of waste into streams, rivers, and oceans. A lot of that waste proceeds right into our supply of water.

We do not always have control over water preservation on a nationwide basis or perhaps a neighborhood basis, however, we can manage how water is utilized in our houses, and there's a lot we may do regarding it. 80% of the water we utilize in our houses is utilized in the restroom. Make sure to take a look at the chapters on the bathroom and kitchen to get some terrific pointers regarding how saving water can conserve money and water.

Chapter 4: Your House

There's a lot you may do where you live to conserve energy via your heating, appliances, the water tank and air-conditioning. Purchasing energy-efficient devices can spare you a lot of cash.

An Energy Star ranked cleaning machine utilizes half the electrical power and water utilized by less effective designs. Cleaning devices utilize approximately 14% of the water consumed in the house. You could spare water by waiting till you have a complete load of clothing to clean. Washers utilize between 32 and 60 gallons of water for every cycle. Approximately 90% of the energy utilized for cleaning clothing goes to warming the water. Here's one thing you may not know - the temperature level of the rinse does not impact the cleansing of the clothing. A cold rinse and a warm water wash are going to work just as effectively as a warm rinse and a warm water wash on almost all clothing.

An Energy Star dishwashing machine may decrease your energy utilization by 30% and spare water as well. You are going to spare much more in case you fill your dishwashing machine prior to running it, while not utilizing the pre-rinse or the heat dry cycles.

Fridges with an energy Star ranking may cut electrical power usage by 15% to 40%. Spare much more energy by letting air flow around the condenser coils in the rear, by examining that the door seals are fastened, and by setting the temperature levels between 35 and 38 ° F and 0 ° F for the freezer. Tidy the condenser coils on the bottom or back of your fridge yearly, at the minimum. Maintain the door gasket tidy to make certain the seal is not broken.

Air conditioning unit - in case all of us raise the settings of our air conditioning unit by 6 °, we might spare 200,000 barrels of oil daily. Do not change your air conditioning unit to a chillier setting when you switch it on. It is not going to cool the space any quicker and it is going to squander energy. Change or clean the filters one time a month; or else the fan works more and takes in more electrical power.

Ovens/stoves - for gas stoves, an electric ignition system is going to utilize around 40% less gas than a pilot light. The pilot burner and light ought to burn with a blue flame. In case the flames yellow, ports and burners are blocked and have to be cleaned up.

Your regional electrical utility is a great source of info regarding energy preservation. They typically offer affordable energy audits, and have literature with pointers regarding energy preservation.

The Kitchen Space

Aside from selecting Energy Star devices, there are lots of things you may do to boost the energy efficiency of your home. A number of these things are relatively simple; it's simply a matter of understanding what they are.

Utilize a Good Detergent

Over 50% of the phosphates in our streams and lakes originate from detergent. Phosphates and other chemicals in our cleaning agents are utilized by makers since they soften water and stop dirt particles from being redeposited on clothing. The issue is the chemicals have adverse effects. As they are cleared into lakes and streams, the fertilized algae expand beyond control. When the algae perish, they decompose and consume the oxygen required by other plans and restore life. The outcome is that the streams and lakes may also perish.

Here are some options:

- Pick a green detergent. There are lots on the marketplace nowadays, so it should not be difficult to find one location - Utilize a detergent developed to operate in cold water. - Stay clear of heavy-duty detergents because they're most likely to have extra chemicals. - Utilize your routine detergent, however, minimize the quantity that you utilize in every wash cycle.

Utilize Green Cleansing Products

You are going to see increasingly more green cleaning items offered to utilize in your house. These are eco-friendly items that do not utilize severe chemicals to do the cleansing. They are constructed out of safe and natural products that clean up effectively without placing any harmful chemicals into our water.

Some individuals utilize nothing but natural cleansing items. These can function as effectively or even better than items you purchase in the shop:

1. Borax is a natural mineral which the disinfectant. It's excellent in the laundry and in the kitchen space, too; it may brighten and bleach your clothes and make them softer.

2. Sodium bicarbonate is a moderate abrasive and functions extremely well as a window cleaner. You may get sodium bicarbonate in volume at hardware shops. Here are several recommendations for usage:

- brighten chrome fittings in kitchen and the restroom with water and baking soda mix.

- tidy worktops appliances and other surfaces using a bit of baking soda on a wet fabric.

- Clean your fridge using 3 tablespoons of baking soda liquified in half a cup of warm water

- tidy your oven by dampening the walls using a wet fabric, spraying baking soda on the surfaces, and leaving it for an hour prior to rubbing it off.

- Soak unclean pans and pots in a warm water basin with a couple of baking soda tablespoons for around an hour. Then tidy them using an abrasive scrubber.

- For coffee or wine spots – before they become dry, put soda water on the stain.

- Utilize baking soda on shower drapes and on mildew in the shower with simply ample water to form it into a paste. Then utilize an old tooth brush to deal with the grout in between the shower tiles.

- Pour half a cup of baking soda down your restroom or kitchen drain, along with a half a cup of vinegar, and after that, a bit of boiling water. This mix dissolves fats that obstruct drains pipes and assists them to remain smelling fresh.

3. Distilled white vinegar removes grease and deodorizers. You may clean up limescale from sinks, showerheads, and tubs, by soaking the showerhead in vinegar, and after that, brushing the line box with an old toothbrush. You may utilize distilled white vinegar to clean the toilet bowl marks or to clean the windows.

4. Lemon juice likewise works on lime on restroom fixtures. If the spots persist, keep the

lemon juice on for a couple of minutes or submerge the tissue in lemon juice and place it on the spot.

Aerate Your Faucets

There's a really easy tool that you may connect to the water faucets in your house to conserve water; it's a low-flow faucet aerator. The typical faucet flow is between 3 and 5 gallons of water per minute with a low flow faucet aerator. You can decrease this flow by half. The incredible thing is that despite the fact that the flow is lowered, it appears more powerful due to the fact that air is being combined with the water.

Setting up these gadgets on bathroom and kitchen sink faucets may cut water use by as high as 280 gallons monthly. For a normal household of 4, it's 3,300 gallons a year for one household. Envision the cost savings if countless households were to utilize these tools. These gadgets are simple to set up. Anybody may do it.

Reusable Containers

Reusable containers are a simple method to reduce paper and plastic wrap use. They are abundant, simple to find, and simple to use for keeping food in your fridge.

Water Heating Units

You may not pay any mind whatsoever to your water heating unit. However, the remarkable reality is that it's the second-largest energy expenditure in the American house. Many individuals maintain their water heating units at 180 °, which is greater than it has to be. This squanders energy by overheating your water, and it likewise reduces the life of the tank. For each 10 ° you turn the water heating unit down, you conserve 6% of the energy utilized.

- Turn your water heating unit to 130 ° - that's sufficiently hot to eliminate germs while still conserving energy.

- Insulate your water heating unit using a blanket produced for water heating units. You may locate these at most hardware shops. This is a particularly great strategy for unheated areas such as the basement. It is going to conserve between 7% and 8% of the energy you have actually been utilizing for that water heating unit.

- Drain approximately 2 quarts of water from the valve faucet situated at the lowest part of the tank every 2 months. This assists to stop the build-up of sediment and it enhances the life and effectiveness of the heating unit.

Ditch the Styrofoam

Styrofoam is created from benzene, which is a recognized carcinogen. It is then transformed to styrene, and after that, created into a foam item. It's non-biodegradable and it is potentially going to be there 500 years from now. It's made up of a fair bit of air, so it uses up a great deal of area. A great deal of the styrofoam finds its way into our oceans and rivers, and it's fatal to marine life. For instance, when sea turtles consume styrofoam, it blocks their systems, and they suffocate.

Simply do not utilize it. From junk food restaurant cups to egg containers, it's simply not safe. Request paper plates and cups.

The Restroom

It was stated previously, however, it bears saying again: approximatel80% of the water we utilize in our houses is utilized in the restroom. This could be correct in some unexpected manners. For example:

- In case you leave the water working as you are brushing your teeth, you're losing between 3 and 5 gallons of water each minute.

- In case you shave with the water running, you're utilizing approximately 10 to 20 gallons every time.

Some basic remedies:

- Brushing your teeth-- rinse and damp your brush to utilize just half a gallon of water.

- Shaving-- in case you fill the basin up, you utilize a gallon of water, that's a reduction of 14 gallons every time you shave.

Showers

If a household of 4 takes five-minute showers every day, they are going to utilize more than 700 gallons of water each week-- that's a three-year drinking water supply for a single person.

A long cozy shower is a luxury a great deal of us do not wish to quit. However, there's a path around that. With a low flow showerhead, you may lower water usage by half. Showers normally represent 32% of house water usage, so by changing the showerhead, you're conserving 16% of overall water use in your house.

Toilets

A genuine surprise here: 40% of the pure water utilized in your home is flushed down the toilet. However, you can easily and rapidly decrease that quantity by almost 40%.

The easiest and most affordable method to do this is via a displacement gadget. You place it in the toilet tank, and it lowers the quantity of water the toilet tank may hold. It may cut your yearly water use by countless gallons, it will not hinder the flush whatsoever, and you are going to never ever see it. Do not utilize a brick for this due to the fact that little pieces can split off and harm your tank. Here's how you make it happen:

- Place a plastic bottle within your toilet tank (a juice or soda bottle are going to function fine).

- Soap off the label, load the bottle with water, and put it in the tank. You may weigh it down with a couple of stones within the bottle.

- Do not let the bottle disrupt the flushing system.

- You may wish to try out various sizes. Various toilets require various quantities of water to preserve the correct pressure for an effective flush. You save 1 to 2 gallons per flush.

You may likewise place a displacement bag in your toilet tank. These are air bags specifically created to displace toilet tank water. You simply fill one with water and hang it on the interior of the tank. Certain utilities offer these free of charge. You may likewise acquire them at plumbing hardware and supply shops. Your save 1 to 2 gallons per flush.

You may likewise set up a toilet dam. It's a gadget that artificially makes your tank tinier. They're offered at plumbing and hardware shops. You would be saving 1 gallon of water per flush.

In case the typical toilet is flushed 8 times daily, that's a reduction between 8 and 16 gallons daily, and 3000 and 5800 gallons yearly.

The Bedroom

Pillowcases and Sheets

A simple method to begin reading your bed room to make it a healthy and tidy comfy retreat is with your pillowcases and sheets and comforter. You need to select natural linen or cotton sheets and natural flannel for the winter season. These are ending up being simple to locate at many of the home items shops.

Stay clear of no iron sheets or petroleum-based polyester sheets due to the fact that the resins in these are harmful and the cleaning does not remove them.

Comforters

Pick a natural alternative for your comforter rather than artificial poly-filled comforters which might are cheaper and less comfy. Search for natural fibers such as natural or goose wool. In case you're allergic to wool, pick natural cotton. These fibers are going to last you a long time.

Pillows

The ideal materials for pillows are natural wool, cotton or latex. Not just are they comfier, however, you are not going to be inhaling hazardous chemicals or pesticides.

Curtains and Drapes

Pick natural linen or cotton for your curtains and drapes to finish your bedroom. Tidy your home using the cleansing items mentioned in this guide to have your green, healthy bedroom.

Chapter 5: Eating Green and Healthy

Food is such a private thing. We delight in it and we treat ourselves with it. However, in case your objective is to live green, there are certain necessary changes to a few of your dietary routines. Initially, here are several stunning stats you may wish to know:

1. In case Americans would decrease their meat consumption by simply 10%, the soybeans and grains conserved would feed 65 million individuals each year.

2. To create 1 pound of beef, we require 16 pounds soybeans and grain, 2600 gallons of water, and the energy equivalent of 1 gallon of fuel.

3. Livestock generation uses up over half of all water consumed in the US.

4. One-third of the North American surface is dedicated to grazing.

5. Cultivating grains, fruits and veggies requires less than 5% as many raw materials as meat generation.

Several easy things you may do today:

- Even if you're a confirmed meat-eater, it is feasible to reduce the quantity of beef you consume.

- Attempt several vegetarian meals. You'd be amazed at how delicious they are, and you are never ever going to know if you never ever attempt.

- Assist your regional farmer's markets. Items that are cultivated locally normally have less pesticide residues than items deliverd from long distances.

A lot of foods on supermarket racks have preservatives and artificial components. You may stay clear of these by checking out labels and selecting items with natural components or by consuming foods fresh from the earth, both veggies and fruits.

Consuming less meat and more veggies has a significant influence on the world since it lowers the quantity of fossil fuel required to create meat and it decreases the quantity of animal waste being created.

Chapter 6: Clothes

Going green with clothes might be tougher for certain people due to the fact that it comes down to purchasing less, yet better quality clothing, using them for longer, and fixing, recycling and repurposing them. That implies purchasing items from natural components made without using chemicals or pesticides.

Purchasing Green Clothes

To purchase green clothes, you need to stay clear of purchasing artificial clothes, although it's highly likely more economical. The most popular artificial components - polyester and nylon - include petrochemicals. Processing them utilizes big quantities of oil, energy, and water in addition to releasing greenhouse gases.

On the other hand, these natural materials are natural and consist of no artificial components:

- Linen is created from flax, which cultivates more quickly than cotton.

- Recycled products are a green option despite the fact that certain chemicals might have entered into their initial generation

- Silk is created from the saliva made by the moth larvae

- Soy produces silk-like, soft items when the leftovers from oil or tofu are refined and spun into fiber.

Looking After Green Clothes

To preserve green clothes, you have to value them sufficient to take fantastic care of them. You can extend the life of your clothes by trading them, donating or keeping them. In each instance, the material of the clothes products requires some attention. Here's how:

- Wash clothing just when they require washing and air dry or line dry.

- Clean clothes from top to bottom - it shields the material.

- Utilize cold water detergent using cold water when you can.

- Pretreat spots instantly

- Remake your clothes into other useful products

In case you have no more usage for a product, do not overlook regifting it. Donating facilities are a good choice, and you are going to be assisting your fellow people and the world.

Chapter 7: Transport

We remain in the middle of a couple of modifications in the vehicle market. Hybrid automobiles are ending up being abundant. Electric automobiles are a possibility. Even diesel is back and much better than it ever has been. The car-buying public is requiring modifications inspired by ecological issues and increasing gas prices. The federal government is enhancing fuel economy requirements, and each car manufacturer is going to need to step up to enhance the effectiveness of their automobiles over the next couple of years.

You might not be trying to find a brand-new automobile today. If not, you can learn how to preserve your existing automobile in the greenest manner possible.

If you're not all set to trade in your present automobile today, here are certain things you may do to boost your automobile's efficiency:

- Have your automobile tuned up. This is the simplest method to make your automobile more fuel-efficient. An inadequately tuned automobile utilizes 10% more gas and releases 10% more poisonous fumes.

- Take note of your gas mileage. This is necessary due to the fact that if there's an unexpected drop in the mileage per gas gallon, you are able to get the issue fixed rapidly.

- Do not allow your vehicle to idle when it's not needed. It requires less gas to begin a vehicle than to keep idling.

- Maintain the fuel filter tidy. Blocked filters squander gas.

- Get rid of unneeded things. Excess weight utilizes gas. An additional hundred pounds are going to reduce your fuel efficiency by more than 1%.

Here's another incredible fact-- if just 100,000 automobile owners frequently tuned up their cars, it would keep 90,000,000 pounds of co2 out of the environment ... Which's less than 1% of the overall drivers in the U.S.

Maintaining the Tires

It may amaze you, however, tires have a huge effect on the environment. When you look after your tires correctly, you save resources and energy, conserve fuel, and decrease the issues associated with tossing them away. Simply, it requires half a petroleum barrel to create the rubber for a single truck tire.

Something you may do today is to maintain your tires inflated. We might conserve as much as 2 billion gas gallons a year with effectively inflated tires.

Radial tires enhance gas mileage, and steel-belted tires are typically the most effective.

Purchase the most fuel-efficient and the longest-lasting tires possible. Ensure your tires are correctly balanced, inflated, and rotated every 8000 miles.

Transportation Alternatives

In case you're an American, you need to confess that we enjoy our vehicles. Much of us own more than one car, and we do not do much to manage them. However, if we truly wish to make a dedication to going green, we need to confess that driving is only one possibility amongst numerous.

Based upon the city in which you reside, you have lots of alternative transportation options -- subways, buses, bikes, trains, or strolling. If you are able to it, even a single day per week would make a huge distinction to the environment.

For example, if just 1% of vehicle owners decided not to drive their vehicles for a single day a week, it would conserve roughly 40 million gallons of gas yearly.

Have you ever considered carpooling? It's a fantastic method to decrease the amount of cars in highway lanes throughout heavy traffic and a fantastic method to lower the quantity of harmful emissions in each urban city. Consult your fellow neighbors and colleagues to find individuals going in the identical direction you are each early morning and night. You may be able to make the most of the high occupancy lanes on the freeway and arrive home quicker every day.

Conclusion

Living green isn't merely about us. It has to do with our future. Our kids' future, and their kids' future. We can decide to go on with our inefficient means, or we can choose that a healthy environment is to be our tradition. It is the most important treasure we can give to our households.

Green living may appear like a pebble contrasted to a stone when it concerns the environment. While, in a way, it is, do not forget that a stack of pebbles accumulates and may eventually dwarf a stone.

I hope that you enjoyed reading through this book and that you have found it useful. If you want to share your thoughts on this book, you can do so by leaving a review on the Amazon page. Have a great rest of the day.

Printed in Great Britain
by Amazon